Healthy On-the-Go

A Guide to Healthier Living for Busy Working Professionals

Kelly Gates & Megan Hill

DISCLAIMER:

The recommendations in this book are not meant to replace the advice given to you by your physician. The information given to you in this book is designed to help you make important decisions about your health, lose weight, and get healthy. Always consult a physician before beginning any diet or exercise program. The authors disclaim any liability directly or indirectly from any use of the material in this book by any person. Mention of specific products or companies or authorities in this book does not imply endorsement by the authors nor does it imply that such companies or authorities endorse this book or authors.

CONTENTS

INTRODUCTION

It's Monday morning and your alarm goes off at 5:30 AM. Here we go – another week of high-stress demands to meet. Feeling like a robot, you get up and go through the motions to get your job done. By the end of the week you feel tired, beat down, and simply warn out.

As weeks go by and demands increase, you start to slip into a "survival mode" way of living. You skip breakfast because you are rushed and by the time lunch rolls around you are starving, so you go out and by a quick and unhealthy meal to satisfy your hunger, and by the end of the day, although you intended to workout, you are completely exhausted and have no energy.

Before you know it, weeks and weeks of this hectic schedule have gone by and you find yourself 20lbs heavier and feeling sick and unhealthy. You begin living off of caffeine and Advil®. When months and years of this type of hectic schedule have passed, you find may yourself struggling with long-term disease, such as cardiovascular disease or metabolic disease, among many other health problems.

Simply put, this lifestyle is not healthy. The choices we all make on a day-to-day basis add up overtime – good or bad. In a culture where healthy living is extremely difficult, we all have to work at it, stay prepared, and be intentional with every decision.

We at **A Stronger Workplace**® have created a step-by-step guide to help you incorporate healthy decisions in every part of your day. Start building these habits into your day and watch your transformation into a healthier, more energized, and happier version of yourself!

So let's go …

CHAPTER 1: GOOD MORNING!

Morning Workouts

The American College of Sports Medicine recommends that adults should get at least 150 minutes of moderate-intensity exercise each week[1]. Exercising in the morning can help you get a jump-start on this recommendation, while energizing you at the start of your day.

Also, exercising in the morning has a multitude of benefits, including that it can improve your sleep quality. Improving sleep quality helps you control your hormones, which helps you manage your weight.

Strive to get at least a few minutes of exercise in the morning. Here are some quick exercise routines based on the time you have available in the morning before you have to jump in the shower:

---

[1] Ewing Garber, C. (2011, July) *ACSM Issues New Recommendations on Quantity and Quality of Exercise*. Retrieved from: http://www.acsm.org/about-acsm/media-room/news-releases/2011/08/01/acsm-issues-new-recommendations-on-quantity-and-quality-of-exercise

If you have 5-10 Minutes, do 1 round.

If you have 10-15 Minutes, do 2 rounds.

If you have 15-20 Minutes, do 3 rounds!

Morning Workout Routine (Beginner):

100 Knees Up (Marching)

10 Modified Push Ups

15 Bodyweight Squats (Modify – Chair Squats)

20 Alternating Lunges

25 Crunches

30 Supermans

50 Small Arm Circles Forward

50 Small Arm Circles Backwards

Morning Workout Routine (Advanced):

100 Jumping Jacks

10 Burpees

15 Bodyweight Squats

20 Push Ups

25 V Ups

100 Jumping Jacks

**Video demonstrations of exercises can be found here:
http://astrongerworkplace.com/videos/

Breakfast Recipes

By starting your day with a healthy breakfast, you will jump start your day with the nutrients and vitamins your body needs, the energy to endure the activities and demands placed on you, as well as kick-start your metabolism to help you manage your weight.

When choosing a breakfast option, go for a balanced meal with carbohydrates, lean protein, and healthy fats. Avoid processed foods and added sugars.

What are healthy fats? We constantly hear about how bad fats are for us, but there are some healthy fats that provide essential nutrients that our bodies crave. Some examples include:

- Avocados
- Nuts and seeds: walnuts, almonds, sunflower and pumpkin seeds
- Olive oil
- Coconut oil
- Chia Seeds
- Nut butters: cashew, almond

Here are some quick and good-for-you breakfast recipes:

Mustard, Avocado, and Dill on a Whole-Wheat English Muffin with Boiled Egg

Ingredients:

2 whole-wheat English muffins, split and toasted

2 teaspoons whole-grain mustard

1 small avocado, sliced

2 hard-boiled eggs

Fresh dill

Directions:

Top the English muffin with the mustard, avocado, and dill, dividing evenly. Serve with the hard-boiled eggs on the side.

Scrambled Eggs with Beans, Pesto, and Tomatoes

Ingredients:

4 large eggs*

3 teaspoons olive oil

½ cup grape tomatoes, halved

½ cup low sodium canned white beans, drained and rinsed

¼ cup store-bought or homemade pesto [see recipe for **homemade pesto****]

4 slices whole-wheat bread, toasted

Directions:

In a medium bowl, beat the eggs with 1 tablespoon of water and ¼ teaspoon each of salt and pepper.

Heat 2 tablespoons of the oil in a large nonstick skillet over medium-high heat. Add the tomatoes and beans; cook, toss occasionally, until warmed through, about 1-2 minutes. Transfer to a plate and wipe the skillet clean. Heat the remaining oil in the skillet and add the eggs. Cook, stirring gently until set but soft, about 1-2 minutes.

Serve the eggs topped with the tomato mixture and pesto, accompanied by the toast.

*Eggs whites can we substituted for the whole eggs.

**The recipe for homemade pesto is in the Lunch Recipes section, under Chicken Pesto Sandwich

---

Avocado Toast

Ingredients:

2 slices whole-wheat or whole-grain bread, toasted

1 avocado, sliced

1 tablespoon olive oil

1 teaspoon fresh lemon juice

1/8 teaspoon red pepper flakes

Kosher or Sea salt

Directions:

Top the bread with the avocado. Mash the avocado gently with a fork. Drizzle with the oil and lemon juice. Sprinkle with ½ teaspoon of salt and the red pepper flakes.

Almond Butter, Yogurt, and Fruit Parfait

Ingredients:

¾ cup plain non-fat Greek yogurt

2 tablespoons almond butter

1 tablespoon local honey

¼ cup halved grapes

3 strawberries, quartered

2 tablespoons chopped roasted almonds

Directions:

The parfait(s) can be made the night before and stored overnight, covered, in the refrigerator for an on-the-go breakfast!

Whisk together the yogurt, almond butter, and honey in a medium bowl until smooth. Combine the fruit and nuts in a medium bowl. Start with a layer of the yogurt mixture in the bottom of a short glass; alternate layers of yogurt with the grapes, strawberries, and roasted almonds.

Morning Pizza

Ingredients:

3 tablespoons low-fat ricotta

1 teaspoon olive oil

4 cherry tomatoes, halved

French baguette or other crusty bread

Dried basil

Freshly ground pepper

Directions:

Slice 2-4 pieces of the crusty bread

Spread the ricotta on each slice

Top the ricotta with the tomato halves

Sprinkle with basil and freshly ground pepper

You can eat them cold or put under the broiler for a few seconds to slightly melt the ricotta and warm the tomatoes.

Strawberry Banana Breakfast Smoothie

Ingredients:

½ cup of frozen strawberries

1 banana

1 cup unsweetened almond or coconut milk

1 Scoop of protein (Garden of Life Raw Vanilla Protein is a recommended brand)

1 Tablespoon of Chia Seeds

1 Cup of Spinach or Kale

Directions:

Mix in blender. Enjoy!

Peanut Butter Overnight Oatmeal

Ingredients:

1/2 cup of gluten-free oats

1 tablespoon chia seeds

2 tablespoons natural salted peanut butter (or almond butter)

1 teaspoon of cinnamon

½ cup unsweetened almond milk

Directions:

Mix all ingredients (except peanut butter) in a Mason jar or bowl. Cover securely and set in refrigerator overnight.

Open the next days, stir in peanut butter, and enjoy!

Overnight oats will keep for up to 2 days, however, they are best in the first 12-24 hours.

TIP: Prepare your breakfasts the night before so they are ready to go the next morning!

CHAPTER 2: MID-DAY SNACKS & EXERCISES

Snacking throughout the day can be a good habit! That is, if those snacks are healthy and nutrient-dense foods. The benefits of snacking include: controlling blood sugar and appetite, improving concentration and mood, increasing metabolism, and maintaining muscle mass.

The best times to snack are mid-morning between breakfast and lunch, and late afternoon between lunch and dinner.

Here are some snack ideas & recipes:

Beet Chips with Curried Yogurt Dip

Ingredients:

1 cup beet chips (Terra® is a good brand)

2 tablespoons plain low-fat Greek yogurt

1/8-1/4 teaspoon curry powder

Directions:

Mix curry powder into the yogurt. Serve with the beet chips.

Crackers with Chocolate-Hazelnut Spread and Banana

Ingredients:

2 crisp bread crackers (Wasa® or Ryvita® are good brands)

1 tablespoon chocolate-hazelnut spread (Nutella® is a good brand)

1 sliced small banana

Directions:

Spread the chocolate-hazelnut spread on the crackers. Top with slices of banana.

Banana, Kale, and Almond Milk Smoothie

Ingredients:

1 medium banana

1 cup chopped kale

1 cup almond milk – unsweetened

Directions:

Put all ingredients in a blender or Nutrabullet® and puree until smooth.

Rice Cake with Peanut Butter, Coconut, and Dried Cherries

Ingredients:

1 rice cake

1 tablespoon peanut butter

2 teaspoons toasted unsweetened shredded coconut

2 teaspoons dried cherries (substitute with dried cranberries)

Directions:

Spread the peanut butter on the rice cake. Sprinkle with the coconut and dried cherries or cranberries.

Whole Grain Bread with Almond Butter and Peaches

Ingredients:

2 teaspoons almond butter

1 slice of toasted whole-grain bred

½ sliced peach

Directions:

Spread the almond butter on the toasted bread. Top with the sliced peaches.

Cherry Tomatoes with Goat Cheese

Ingredients:

5 large cherry tomatoes, halved

2 tablespoons fresh goat cheese

2 teaspoons chopped herbs (such as chives, basil, or parsley)

Directions:

Top the halved tomatoes with the goat cheese. Sprinkle the chopped herbs on top.

Roasted Edamame with Sea Salt and Black Pepper

Ingredients:

16 oz. frozen shelled edamame

2 teaspoons extra virgin olive oil

1 teaspoon sea salt

½ teaspoon freshly ground black pepper

Directions:

Preheat oven to 375*. Rinse the edamame under warm water for a few seconds to melt any ice crystals. Spread the edamame on a clean dish towel and pat gently to remove excess water. In a mixing bowl, toss the edamame with the olive oil, salt, and pepper. Spread the edamame in a single layer on a sheet pan and roast for 30-40 minutes, stirring every 10 minutes. Watch for the edamame to begin puffing and turning golden-brown. Remove the pan from the oven, transfer the edamame to a serving bowl or let cool, and store in an airtight container.

Pecan Pie Granola

Ingredients:

½ cup chopped pecans

½ cup chopped almonds

1 ½ cups old fashioned oats

¼ cup stevia

½ teaspoon salt

2 teaspoons cinnamon

½ teaspoon pumpkin pie spice

2 tablespoons maple syrup

1 egg white

Directions:

Mix ingredients together. Spread on baking sheet. Bake at 375* for 30 minutes. Store in airtight container.

Mid-Day Desk Stretches & Exercises:

Our bodies are not designed to sit for long periods of time. It is important to stay active throughout your day as much as possible. Taking short walks on your breaks and engaging in exercises and stretches at your desk can be very helpful!

Here are some Desk Stretches and Exercises to try. Choose 2 or 3 and perform them every 1-2 hours.

Arm Circles

Calf Raises

Chair Dips

Chest stretch

Chair Squats

Cradle stretch

Desk Push Ups

Hamstring Stretch

Lateral Raises

Lat Stretch

Leg Swings

Quad Stretch

Shoulder Stretch

Tricep Stretch

Spinal Twist

CHAPTER 3: LUNCH & LUNCHTIME EXERCISES

We encourage you to start bringing your lunch to work! Not only will you decrease your waistline, but you will save money! Bring leftovers from dinner the night before, or try some of these wonderful Lunch Recipes:

Avocado Chicken Salad

Ingredients:

2 cups shredded, cooked white meat chicken

1 avocado, chopped

½ teaspoon garlic powder

½ teaspoon salt

½ teaspoon pepper

2 teaspoons lime juice

1 teaspoon fresh cilantro

¼ cup light mayonnaise

¼ cup plain low fat Greek yogurt

To serve: choose from pita pocket, crackers, or lettuce

Directions:

Mix all ingredients in a large bowl. Cover and refrigerate for 20-30 minutes to let the flavors blend together. Serve in a pita pocket or with crackers, or on a bed of lettuce. Can make the night/day before and pack in a lunch container.

Cowboy Caviar

Ingredients:

1 can low sodium black beans, drained and rinsed

1 can low sodium yellow corn, drained and rinsed or 1 ½ cups fresh corn kernels

3 Roma tomatoes, diced

2 diced avocados

¼ cup red onion, diced

¼ cup cilantro, finely chopped

Juice of 1 lime

½ teaspoon salt

½ cup low sodium Italian dressing

To serve: choose from: pita pocket, crackers, lettuce

Directions:

Sprinkle the lime juice on the avocado so it doesn't brown quickly. Combine all ingredients in a large mixing bowl. Cover and refrigerate for an hour to marinate the flavors together. Although this salad is best served the same day you make it, it will still be good the next day even with the avocados turning a bit brown. Pack in a sealed container to take to work. Serve on a bed of lettuce or in a pita pocket or with crackers – or just eat it plain like a salad.

Sweet and Sour Broccoli Salad

Ingredients:

½ cup sweet and sour sauce

3 small stalks of broccoli, cleaned, blanched, and cut into small florets

1 tablespoon sesame oil

Sesame seeds

Handful of roasted cashews

2 stalks of sliced green scallions

Directions:

Pour half of the sweet and sour sauce in a mixing bowl. Add the broccoli and mix together, coating evenly with the sauce. Drizzle the sesame oil and mix together. Toss in the sesame seeds and more sweet and sour sauce. Toss in the cashews and mix together. Top with the scallions. Pack in a sealed container to take to work.

Spinach, Pasta, and Chickpea Soup

Ingredients:

1 tablespoon extra virgin olive oil

3 garlic cloves, thinly sliced

2 green onions, thinly sliced

4 cups fat free, low sodium chicken broth

2 cups water

¾ cup uncooked orzo

1 tablespoon grated lemon zest/rind

1 15-ounce can no-salt-added chickpeas (garbanzo beans), drained and rinsed

1 tablespoon lemon juice

½ teaspoon freshly ground black pepper

1/8 teaspoon salt

1 tablespoon chopped fresh oregano

1 6-ounce package fresh baby spinach

1/3 cup grated Parmesan cheese

Directions:

Heat a large saucepan, add the olive oil to the pan. Add the garlic and onions to the olive oil, sauté for about 30 seconds until fragrant. Add chicken broth and 2 cups water, bring to a boil. Add orzo, lemon rind/zest, and chickpeas. Cover and cook for 10-15 minutes or until the orzo is done. Add the oregano, lemon juice, pepper, salt, and spinach. Let the spinach wilt. When the soup has cooled, put into individual sealed containers to take to work and refrigerate. Serve with some of the Parmesan cheese sprinkled on top.

For a vegetarian version, substitute veggie broth for the chicken broth.

Spicy Tomato and White Bean Soup

Ingredients:

1 14-ounce can fat-free, low sodium chicken broth

2 teaspoons chili powder

1 teaspoon ground cumin

1 16-ounce can navy beans, drained and rinsed

1 medium Poblano chile, halved and seeded

½ medium yellow onion, cut into ½-inch thick wedges

1 pint grape tomatoes

¼ cup chopped fresh cilantro

2 tablespoons fresh lime juice

1 tablespoon extra virgin olive oil

½ teaspoon sale

Fresh cilantro sprigs, optional

Directions:

Combine 1 cup of the chicken broth, chili powder, cumin, and beans in a large pot or Dutch oven over medium-high heat. Bring to a boil. Combine the remaining broth, Poblano chile, and onion in a food processor, pulsing until the vegetables are finely chopped. Add this onion mixture to the soup pot. Put the tomatoes and chopped cilantro in the food processor, and pulse until coarsely chopped. Add this tomato mixture to the soup pot. Bring to a boil. Cover, reduce heat, and simmer for 5 minutes or until the veggies are tender. Remove from heat and let cool. Put into individual sealed containers to take to work and refrigerate. Garnish with the cilantro sprigs, if desired.

For a vegetarian version, substitute veggie broth for the chicken broth.

Kale Salad with Cranberry Vinaigrette

Ingredients:

3 tablespoons extra virgin olive oil

1 shallot, peeled and thinly sliced

3 cloves garlic, coarsely chopped

1 cup dried cranberries

2 tablespoons red wine vinegar

2 teaspoons honey

Juice and rind/zest of ½ lemon

1/8 teaspoon salt

1/8 teaspoon black pepper

1 bunch kale, thick stems removed and very thinly sliced

¼ cup sliced almonds

¼ cup crumbled blue cheese or goat cheese, optional

Directions:

Cranberry Vinaigrette: Heat 2 tablespoons of olive oil in a sauté pan, add the shallots and garlic and cook until fragrant and tender. Turn off the heat. Add the cranberries, red wine vinegar, honey, and lemon juice and rind/zest. Stir to combine. Season with salt and pepper.

Salad: In a large bowl, toss the kale with remaining olive oil and an extra pinch of salt. Massage the kale gently to combine.

Put the salad in individual sealed containers to take to work and refrigerate. Put the almonds in a baggie – also the cheese, if you want to include it. Put the vinaigrette into a sports bottle so you can dress your salad when you're ready to eat it. This way, the salad won't be soggy and the kale will be crisp. Add the almonds and optional cheese when you pour on the vinaigrette.

Chicken Pesto Sandwich

Ingredients:

2 cups cooked, shredded chicken breast

¼ cup fat free plain Greek yogurt

Kosher salt and freshly ground black pepper, to taste

1 baguette, cut into 3-4 equal pieces

2 cups arugula, for serving

2 Roma tomatoes, thinly sliced, for serving

8 ounces Mozzarella cheese, sliced

1 cup fresh basil leaves

3 cloves garlic, peels

3 tablespoons pine nuts

1/3 cup grated Parmesan cheese

1/3 cup extra virgin olive oil

If you prefer, you can use store-bought pesto. If so, eliminate the ingredients after the Mozzarella cheese.

Directions:

For the pesto: Combine the basil, garlic, pine nuts, and Parmesan in a food processor. Add salt and pepper to taste. With the processor running, add the olive oil in a slow stream until emulsified. Set aside.

In a large bowl, combine chicken, ½ cup pesto, Greek yogurt, and salt and pepper to taste.

For serving: Spread some of the remaining pesto on the bread, add the arugula, tomatoes, and sliced mozzarella. Top with the chicken pesto mixture. To take to work, build the sandwich and put in an airtight baggie or container.

Quinoa Avocado Salad

Ingredients:

2 cups of quinoa

1 large cucumber

2 roma tomatoes

1 bunch of green onions

1 green bell pepper

1 avocado

Salt

Pepper

Balsamic vinaigrette dressing

Directions:

Cook quinoa and then place in large bowl and refrigerate.

Chop up cucumber, tomatoes, green onions, bell pepper, and avocado into small pieces and add to large bowl of Quinoa and mix well.

Add salt, pepper, and balsamic vinaigrette to taste.

Serving: This salad is great with chicken or as a side dish. This recipe can be pre-made ahead of time during meal prep and divided up into small containers (make sure to seal tight to keep avocados fresh) to take to work.

Lunch Time Workouts

Try your best to take a full hour for lunch. Use it to eat and then recharge your batteries with a walk or by doing this quick 12 Minute HIIT (High Intensity Interval Training) Workout:

Lunch Time Workout (Beginner)

TABATA (8 Rounds of Each Exercise, 20 Seconds Exercise, 10 Seconds Rest)

Exercise 1: Bodyweight Squats (Modify to Char Squats if needed)

Exercise 2: Modified Tricep Dips

Exercise 3: Leg Lifts

Lunch Time Workout (Advanced)

TABATA (8 Rounds of Each Exercise, 20 Seconds Exercise, 10 Seconds Rest)

Exercise 1: Squat Jumps

Exercise 2: Push Ups

Exercise 3: V-Ups

---

*Did you know....*High-intensity interval training (HIIT) can boost metabolism and accelerate weight loss. During HIIT, a person consumes more oxygen than in slower, distance exercise, which can increase post-exercise metabolism. Research has shown one session of HIIT can burn calories for 1.5 - 24 hours after exercise[2]

---

[2] Bracko, M. (2011, August) *For All-Day Metabolism Boost, Try Interval Training.* Retrieved from: http://www.acsm.org/about-acsm/media-room/acsm-in-the-news/2011/08/01/for-all-day-metabolism-boost-try-interval-training

CHAPTER 4: DINNER & EVENING WORKOUT

Here are some healthy and family-friendly dinner recipes:

Chicken and Pasta Primavera

Ingredients:

1   9oz package of fettuccine pasta, plain or wheat or spinach

2 Medium carrots, thinly sliced lengthwise

1 Medium zucchini, halved lengthwise and thinly sliced lengthwise

¾ cup frozen whole kernel corn

12 ounces deli-roasted chicken cut into ½-inch strips (about 2 ½ cups)

1 ½ cups chicken broth

4 teaspoons cornstarch

1 tablespoon snipped fresh tarragon or basil – or use dried if you don't have fresh

1 ½ teaspoons finely shredded lemon zest

½ cup sour cream – light

2 tablespoons Dijon mustard

Directions:

Cook the pasta according to package directions, adding the carrots, zucchini, and corn to the water with the pasta. Drain the pasta and veggies when cooked to al dente. Return it all to the pan and add the chicken.

In another saucepan, combine chicken broth, cornstarch, lemon zest, and tarragon or basil. Cook and stir over medium heat until thickened and bubbly. Cook and stir for 2 minutes more. Remove from heat. Stir in the sour cream and mustard. Pour over the pasta and veggies to coat; gently toss. Serve immediately.

This recipe warms well for leftovers or an easy lunch the next day.

Peach-Mustard Glazed Ham

Ingredients:

2 tablespoons brown sugar

2 tablespoons spicy brown mustard

1/3 cup peach or apricot nectar

1 pound cooked ham slice, cut into ¾ to 1 inch thick

4 medium peaches, peeled and halved lengthwise

2 small green and/or red sweet peppers, each cut crosswise into 4 rings

Directions:

For the glaze, in a bowl combine the sugar and mustard. Gradually whisk in the nectar until smooth.

To prevent the ham from curling, make shallow cuts around the edge at 1-inch intervals. Brush one side of the ham with the glaze.

Grill the ham glazed-side down or bake it glazed-side up in the oven. Turn the ham over and add more glaze to the unglazed side. Add the peaches and peppers to the pan or grill. Brush the ham, peaches, and peppers with more glaze. Cook/grill until everything is heated through.

Sun-dried Tomato Burgers

Ingredients:

1 pound lean ground beef

1 tablespoon finely chopped, drained, oil-packed sun-dried tomatoes

1 teaspoon finely shredded lemon or lime peel/zest

½ teaspoon salt

¼ teaspoon black pepper

¼ cup light mayonnaise

2 tablespoons snipped fresh basil

1 fresh jalapeno pepper, seeded and finely chopped

Buns or rolls for the hamburgers – 4

1 cup lightly packed arugula or baby spinach leaves

Directions:

In a medium bowl, combine the beef, tomatoes, lemon/lime zest, salt, and pepper. Mix well. Shape into four patties. Grill the patties until meat is no longer pink in the middle.

Meanwhile, in a small bowl, combine the mayo, basil, and jalapeno. Toast the buns, cut sides down, if desired – spread a little olive oil or butter on the buns to assist with toasting.

Put the cooked patties on the bottom buns, top with the mayo mixture and arugula or baby spinach.

Jalapeno handling tip: When handling fresh jalapeno or other fresh chili peppers, wear rubber gloves to prevent potential skin burns. The knife and cutting service of the board will have residual juice from the pepper, so be sure to clean both thoroughly before using on other food items.

Lemony Flank Steak

This recipe requires a 2-hour or overnight marinade. Easy to do this the night before and it's ready to cook for dinner the next day.

Ingredients:

1 ½ pound beef flank steak or boneless top sirloin steak

1 teaspoon finely shredded lemon peel/zest

½ cup lemon juice

2 tablespoons sugar

2 tablespoons soy sauce

2 teaspoons fresh oregano or ½ teaspoon dried oregano

¼ teaspoon pepper

Lemon slices

Fresh oregano leaves (optional)

Directions:

Trim fat from the steak. Score it on both sides by making shallow cuts at 1-inch intervals in diamond pattern. Place the steak in a plastic bag set in a shallow dish to marinade.

For the marinade: combine the lemon peel/zest, lemon juice, sugar, soy sauce, oregano, and pepper. Pour into the bag to coat the steak. Marinate in refrigerator for at least 2 hours or overnight.

Drain the steak, but reserve the marinade. Grill the steak on an uncovered grill over medium heat until desired doneness, turning and brushing with the marinade.

To serve, thinly slice the steak diagonally, across the grain. Garnish with lemon slices and fresh oregano.

Black and White Bean Chili

This recipe is vegetarian and makes for great leftovers for lunch or dinner the next day.

Ingredients:

1 medium onion, chopped

1 clove garlic, minced

1 tablespoon olive oil

15 oz. can white kidney or cannellini beans, rinsed and drained

15 oz. can black beans, rinsed and drained

14 ½ oz. can vegetable broth

1 cup chopped, peeled jicama or potato

4 oz. can diced green chili peppers

1 teaspoon ground cumin

2 tablespoons fresh cilantro (you can leave out this ingredient if you don't like cilantro)

1 tablespoon lime juice

¼ cup crumbled Queso Fresco or feta cheese (1 oz.)

Directions:

In a large saucepan, cook the onion and garlic in the oil until tender. Stir in the white beans and black beans, along with the broth, jicama/potato, green chili peppers, and cumin.

Bring to a boil, reduce heat, simmer – covered – for about 10 minutes, until jicama/potato is tender. Stir in the cilantro – if desired – and lime juice and heat through.

Ladle into soup bowls and top each with the cheese.

Italian Greens and Cheese Tortellini Soup

This recipe is vegetarian.

Ingredients:

1 ½ cup finely chopped onion

5 cloves garlic, minced

1 teaspoon dried Italian herbs seasoning, crushed

1 tablespoon olive oil

14 ½ oz. cans (2 of them) or 3 ½ cups reduced-sodium vegetable broth

1 ½ cups water

9 oz. package fresh or frozen cheese-filled tortellini pasta

2 cups sugar snap peas, strings and tips removed, and halved crosswise

2 cups shredded spinach

2 teaspoons lemon juice

2 tablespoons finely shredded Parmesan cheese

Directions:

In a large pot or Dutch oven, cook the onion, garlic, and Italian herb seasoning in the oil over medium heat until the onion is tender. Add the broth and water. Bring to a boil then add the tortellini. Return to a boil, reduce heat, and simmer – uncovered – for about 5 minutes.

Stir in the snap peas, spinach and lemon juice. Return to a boil, reduce heat, and simmer – uncovered – for 2 more minutes.

Ladle into soup bowls. Top each with the Parmesan cheese.

Mediterranean Couscous Salad

This recipe is vegetarian.

Ingredients:

For the Couscous:

1 cup couscous

1 medium red sweet pepper, chopped

½ cup chopped cucumber

¼ cup sliced or chopped pitted Kalamata olives

¼ cup crumbled feta cheese (1 oz.)

For the Lemon-Oregano Vinaigrette:

3 tablespoons lemon juice

2 tablespoons olive oil

1 tablespoon fresh oregano or ¾ teaspoon dried oregano

1 tablespoon fresh mint or ¼ teaspoon dried mint

For the Pita Chips:

2 pita bread rounds, cut in half then cut each half into 6 wedges

½ teaspoon garlic salt

Directions:

For the Couscous:

Cook the couscous according to package directions. Fluff with a fork before adding other ingredients.

Put the fluffed couscous in a bowl, drizzle the Lemon-Oregano Vinaigrette. Let it cool for 10 minutes, then add the red pepper, cucumber, and olives. Toss to combine. Sprinkle with the cheese. Serve with the pita chips.

For the Lemon-Oregano Vinaigrette:

In a screw-top jar or tightly covered bowl, combine all the vinaigrette ingredients and shake well.

For the Pita Chips:

Arrange wedges in a single layer on a greased baking sheet. Brush with olive oil or coat with nonstick cooking spray. Sprinkle with the garlic salt. Bake at 400 degrees for 6-8 minutes or until crisp and lightly browned.

Grilled Tuna with Wilted Spinach

This marinade requires only 5-10 minutes of soaking time.

Ingredients:

1 ¼ pounds fresh skinless tuna fillet or 4 serving-size portions, about ¾ inch thick

For the marinade:

3 tablespoons balsamic vinegar

1 tablespoon olive oil

¼ teaspoon salt

¼ teaspoon garlic pepper

1 medium red onion, cut into ¼ inch slices

6 cups baby spinach or torn spinach or mixed salad greens

2 cups grape tomatoes or cherry tomatoes, halved

2 tablespoons water

Directions:

Rinse fish, pat dry. Cut fish into serving size portions, if you have a single hunk of fish.   Lightly sprinkle with salt and pepper, place in a shallow dish. Cover and marinade at room temperature for 5-10 minutes. Drain the fish, but reserve the marinade.

For the Marinade:

In a small bowl, stir together the vinegar, oil, ¼ teaspoon salt, and garlic pepper.

After fish has soaked, grill the fish on an uncovered grill over medium heat until the fish flakes easily with a fork and the onion is tender. Turn and brush the fish with the marinade.

While the fish is cooking, in a large skillet, combine and toss together the spinach, tomatoes, and water. Cook for 3-4 minutes until the spinach begins to wilt, stirring occasionally. Transfer the spinach mixture to a serving platter and top with the fish and onion slices. Drizzle with the remaining vinegar mixture.

Chicken with Mango Chutney

This chutney features mangoes and is ready in less than 10 minutes

Ingredients:

1 ripe mango, seeded, peeled, and sliced

¼ cup dried currants, cranberries, or raisins

¼ cup thinly sliced green onions

2-3 tablespoons cider vinegar

2 tablespoons brown sugar

½ teaspoon mustard seed, crushed – or ¼ teaspoon dried mustard

1/8 teaspoon sale

1 pound skinless, boneless chicken thighs

1 teaspoon Chinese five-spice powder

Directions:

NOTE: Mangoes have oval, flattish pits. When slicing, keep this in mind.

In a medium saucepan, combine half the mango slices, currants/cranberries/raisins, green onions, vinegar, brown sugar, mustard, and salt. Bring to a boil, reduce heat, simmer – covered – for 5 minutes. Remove from heat.

Chop the remaining mango slices and set aside. Rub the chicken with the five-spice powder. Grill uncovered over medium heat for 10-12 minutes, or bake in the oven until cooked through.

To serve, stir the chopped mango into the cooked mango mixture. Serve with the chicken.

Southwest Chicken Salad with Grilled Oranges

This salad can be made as an entree or a smaller version can be made as a side salad by omitting the chicken.

Ingredients:

½ cup bottled poppy seed salad dressing

1 small fresh jalapeno pepper, seeded and finely chopped

½ teaspoon finely shredded orange peel/zest

4 medium boneless, skinless chicken breasts

2 oranges, peeled and sliced to ½ inch thick

1 red sweet pepper, quartered

8 cups torn mixed salad greens

1 small jicama, peeled and cut into thin bite-size strips

Directions:

In a small bowl, combine the salad dressing, jalapeno, and orange peel/zest. Take our 1 tablespoon of the dressing mixture and set aside. Brush the chicken, orange slices, and red pepper wedges with that 1 tablespoon of dressing.

Grill the chicken, orange slices, and red pepper on an uncovered grill over medium heat for 12-15 minutes until chicken is fully cooked, or bake in the oven until the chicken is fully cooked.

When done, transfer the chicken, oranges, and peppers to a cutting board and cut the chicken and peppers into bite-size strips; quarter the orange slices.

Meanwhile, in a large mixing bowl, toss together the jicama and salad greens. Add the chicken, oranges, and sweet peppers, drizzle with the dressing mixture. Season to taste with black pepper.

Post Workout/Evening Stretching Routine

Flexibility is a component of physical fitness that is often overlooked. Stretching will help you move easier without discomfort, reduce your risk of injury, and reduce stress. Finish your day with this 10-Minute Stretch Routine:

- Standing Straddle – 20 Seconds Each Side/Middle
- Quad Stretch – 20 Seconds Each Leg
- Hip Flexor/Hamstring Stretch – 20 Seconds Each Position/Each Leg
- Straddle Stretch – 20 Seconds Each Side/Middle
- Pike Stretch – 20 Seconds
- Figure 4 Stretch – 20 Seconds Each Leg
- Trunk Twist – 20 Seconds Each Side
- Seal/Cat Stretch – 20 Seconds Each
- Achilles Stretch – 20 Seconds

CHAPTER 5: SLOW COOKER RECIPES

Slow cookers can help you save time in the kitchen and make cooking an easy process. Throw your meal together in your slow cooker first thing in the morning and have your meal ready for you when you arrive home from work. Here are some of our favorite recipes:

NOTE: Slow cookers vary in how they cook and by their size. You may need to adjust ingredient quantities if you have a small slow-cooker. These recipes are for a 6-quart slow-cooker.

Mediterranean Roast Turkey

Serve this slow cooker roast with mashed sweet potatoes.

Slow cooker time: 7.5 hours total

Ingredients:

2 cups chopped onion

½ cup pitted Kalamata olives

½ cup julienne-cut, drained, oil-packed sun dried tomatoes

2 tablespoons lemon juice

1 ½ teaspoons minced garlic

1 teaspoon Greek seasoning mix (McCormick's is a good brand)

½ teaspoon salt

¼ teaspoon freshly ground black pepper

4 pounds boneless, skinless turkey breast – trimmed

½ cup fat-free, lower sodium chicken broth, divided

3 tablespoons all-purpose flour

Thyme sprigs (optional)

Directions:

Combine the first 9 ingredients in an electric slow cooker. Add ¼ cup of chicken broth. Cover and cook on low for 7 hours.

Combine the remaining chicken broth and flour in a small bowl; stir with a whisk until smooth. Add this broth mixture to the slow cooker. Cover and cook on low for another 30 minutes. Cut turkey into slices for serving.

Slow-Simmered Meat Sauce with Pasta

You can choose whichever dried pasta you prefer for this sauce recipe.

Slow-cooker time: 8.5 hours total

Ingredients:

16 oz. uncooked pasta of your choice

1 tablespoon olive oil

2 cups chopped onion

1 cup chopped carrots

6 garlic cloves, minced

8 oz. of hot Italian sausage links with casings removed

1 pound ground sirloin

½ cup Kalamata olives, pitted and sliced

¼ cup no-salt-added tomato paste

1 ½ teaspoons sugar

1 teaspoon Kosher salt

½ teaspoon crushed red pepper

28 oz. can no-salt-added crushed tomatoes, undrained

1 cup no-salt-added tomato sauce

1 tablespoon chopped fresh oregano (or ¼ tablespoon dried oregano)

½ cup torn fresh basil, if desired

3 oz. shaved fresh Parmigiano-Reggiano cheese

Directions:

Heat a pan over medium-high heat. Add the oil to the pan and sauté the onions and carrots for about 4 minutes. Add the garlic and sauté for 1 minute more. Put this veggie mixture in the slow cooker. Add the sausage and beef to the skillet, sauté them for 6 minutes or until browned, stirring to crumble. Remove the meat mixture from the pan with a slotted spoon and place the mixture on a layer of paper towels to absorb excess grease. Then add the meat to the slow-cooker, stir in the olives and the next 6 ingredients (through the tomato sauce). Cover and cook on low for 8 hours.

Stir the oregano into the cooked sauce.

Cook pasta according to package directions.   Serve the sauce over the pasta.

Provençal Chicken Supper

Use bone-in chicken breasts for this French-country dish

Slow-cooker time: 8 hours

Ingredients:

4 chicken breast halves, skinned and bone-in

2 teaspoons dried basil

1/8 teaspoon salt

1/8 teaspoon freshly ground black pepper

1 cup diced yellow bell pepper

15.5 oz. can cannellini beans or other white beans, rinsed and drained

14.5 oz. can diced tomatoes with basil, garlic, and oregano, undrained

Basil sprigs (optional)

Directions:

Place the chicken in the slow cooker; sprinkle with salt and pepper and dried basil. Add the bell pepper, beans, and tomatoes. Cover and cook on low for 8 hours.

Slow Cooker Brisket Sandwiches

Serve on brioche buns (or another of your favorite buns) with coleslaw

Slow cooker time: 8 hours

Ingredients:

2 tablespoons vegetable oil

1 five or six pound brisket, cut into 3 pieces

Kosher salt and freshly ground black pepper

4 cloves of garlic, smashed and peeled

12 oz. bottle stout beer

4 stalks of celery, cut into large pieces

2/3 cup packed dark brown sugar

½ cup tomato paste

½ cup red wine vinegar

1/3 cup Dijon mustard

1/3 cup soy sauce

2 bay leaves

1 teaspoon paprika

Brioche or other rolls, split open and toasted

Coleslaw, for serving (this can be store-bought or homemade)

Directions:

Heat the veggie oil in a skillet, season the brisket with salt and pepper, and brown it on all sides, about 10 minutes, adding the garlic in the last 2 minutes. Transfer the meat and garlic to the slow cooker. Pour the beer into the skillet and simmer for 30 seconds, scraping up the browned bits from the pan; add the beer mixture to the slow cooker.

Nestle the celery around the meat and add the brown sugar, tomato paste, vinegar, mustard, soy sauce, bay leaves, and paprika. Stir together then cover and cook on low for 8 hours, or on high for 6 hours. When done, transfer the meat to a cutting board and let it rest for 10 minutes. Then thinly slice.

Serve open-face on the toasted brioche with the coleslaw either below or on top of the meat, drizzled with the cooking liquid.

Pesto & Sundried Tomato Chicken Pasta or Quinoa

Serve over pasta or quinoa.

Slow Cooker Time: 8 hours

Ingredients:

1 3oz package of sun dried tomatoes

1/3 cup chicken broth

1 teaspoon dried basil leaves

1 onion, chopped

3 cloves garlic, minced

½ teaspoon salt

1/8 teaspoon pepper

2 Cups baby spinach leaves

4 boneless, skinless chicken breasts

Directions:

Add all ingredients to slow cooker. Cook on low for 8 hours. Serve over pasta or rice. Enjoy!

Slow Cooker BBQ Chicken

Ingredients:

4 boneless, skinless chicken breasts

1 ½ cups BBQ sauce

1 tablespoon worcestershire sauce

¼ cup chicken broth.

Salt to taste

Directions:

Season chicken breast lightly with a small pinch of sea salt. Put in slow cooker.

In a mixing bowl combine BBQ sauce, Worcestershire sauce, and chicken broth. Stir until well combined.

Pour over chicken and cook on HIGH for 3-4 hours.

Shred with fork and then serve on buns, over rice, in wraps, or eat as is!

CHAPTER 6: GUILT-FREE SWEET TREATS

We all need a sweet treat from time to time! Don't be afraid to treat yourself, particularly after a hard day at work.   Here are some better-for-you options to satisfy that sweet tooth:

Almond Butter Coconut Chia Seed Bites

Ingredients:

2 tablespoons coconut oil, melted

3 tablespoons natural almond butter

1 tablespoon chia seeds

2 tablespoons shredded coconut

1 teaspoon pine nuts

2 tablespoons unsweetened cocoa powder

¼ teaspoon almond extract

Directions:

Combine all ingredients and mix well. Chill in the refrigerator for 30 minutes. Remove the mixture and roll into bite-sized pieces. Roll in additional shredded coconut, if desired. Put back in the refrigerator for another 10 minutes.

Dark Chocolate Avocado Truffles

Ingredients:

6 oz. dark chocolate (70% or higher)

½ cup mashed avocado

¼ teaspoon vanilla extract

Pinch of salt

2 tablespoons cocoa powder (for rolling) – optional

Directions:

Combine the chocolate, vanilla extract, and pinch of salt over a double boiler, melt until completely smooth. Turn off the heat.   Note: If you don't have a double boiler, you can use a heat-safe glass/ceramic mixing bowl over a saucepan.

Mash the avocado with a fork until there are no lumps, then stir it into the melted chocolate mixture until smooth and thickened. Put the mixture in the refrigerator to set for about 20 minutes, or until slightly firm to the touch. Roll into bite-size balls in the palm of your hand. Roll in the loose cocoa powder, if desired. Store in the refrigerator.

Pineapple-Raspberry Parfaits

Ingredients:

2 eight-oz. containers (2 cups) non-fat peach yogurt

½ pint fresh raspberries (about 1 ¼ cups)

1 ½ cups fresh, frozen, or canned pineapple chunks

Directions:

Divide and layer the yogurt, raspberries, and pineapple into four high-ball glasses. Serve.

Cherries with Ricotta and Toasted Almonds

Ingredients:

¾ cup frozen pitted cherries

2 tablespoons part-skim ricotta

1 tablespoon toasted slivered almonds

Directions:

Heat the cherries in the microwave on high until warm, about 1-2 minutes. Top the cherries with ricotta and sprinkle with the almonds. Serve.

Cinnamon Streusel Crisps

This recipe requires frozen sugar cookie dough, so remember to work this into your prep time.

Ingredients:

One 16.5 oz. package refrigerated sugar cookie dough

¼ cup packed light brown sugar

¼ cup finely chopped pecans

¾ teaspoon ground cinnamon

¼ teaspoon ground nutmeg (optional)

Directions:

Freeze the sugar cookie dough 1 hour before using.

Preheat oven to 350°; place rack in center of oven.

Remove the cookie dough from the freezer and place on a cutting board. Slice into ¼-inch slices and arrange 2 inches apart on 2 parchment paper-lined baking sheets.

Combine the brown sugar, chopped pecans, cinnamon, and nutmeg in a small mixing bowl. Top the cookies with ¾ teaspoon each of the mixture. Bake for 12 minutes or until cookie edges are crisp and browned. Let cool for about 3 minutes on the baking sheet, then move to a wire rack to cool completely.

Frozen Banana Pops

Ingredients:

1 ripe banana

4 popsicle sticks

3 oz. vanilla soy yogurt (or dairy yogurt, if desired)

1/8 cup mini chocolate chips (Ghirardelli is a good brand)

Directions:

Line a small cutting board or plate with parchment paper

Peel the banana

Cut it in half, then cut the halves in half, to make four pieces

Push a popsicle stick ¾ of the way through the bottom of each piece

Dip each piece in the yogurt, twirling it around to coat evenly

Sprinkle the chocolate chips onto a plate and roll the banana pieces in them to coat.

Place in the freezer for at least 4 hours.

Brown Rice Crispy Treats

The marshmallow cream from the traditional crispy treat recipe is replaced with honey (or brown rice syrup); almond butter and coconut oil replace the butter.

Ingredients:

2/3 cup honey (or brown rice syrup, if you have it)

¼ cup almond butter

1 tablespoon coconut oil

½ teaspoon vanilla extract

Pinch of salt

4 cups of brown rice crisp cereal

2 tablespoons of mini chocolate chips (Ghirardelli is a good brand)

Directions:

Put the brown rice cereal in a large mixing bowl.

Combine the honey (or brown rice syrup), almond butter, and coconut oil in a sauce pan over medium heat. Stir until mixture is combined and creamy. Remove from heat, add the vanilla and the salt.

Pour the honey mixture over the brown rice cereal and mix well until combined. Press this mixture into a square baking dish lined with parchment paper, then press the chocolate chips into the top.

Let cool in the refrigerator for 1 hour before cutting into squares.

Chocolate-Peanut Butter Energy Bites

Ingredients:

1 cup (dry) oatmeal

½ cup chocolate chips

½ cup peanut butter

½ cup ground flaxseed

1/3 cup honey

1 teaspoon vanilla

Directions:

Mix ingredients together in a large bowl. Roll into bit size balls. Refrigerate to set.

Strawberry – Banana Ice Cream

Ingredients:

3 ripe frozen bananas

1 cup frozen strawberries

½ teaspoon vanilla extract

½ cup almond milk

Directions:

Mix ingredients in blender food processor until creamy. Serve immediately.

CHAPTER 7: STAYING HEALTHY WHILE TRAVELING

Busy business people often have to travel for work, particularly if you are in a sales role. Sometimes we spend more time on the road than we do at home. But, don't let your exercise and healthful eating routines fall apart while you're traveling from point A to point B to point C and home again. Here are some easy-to-follow and remember tips to take with you ...

Food:

- Bring a refillable water bottle. You can fill it after you're through airport security. And you can take it with you to all your meetings, in the car, etc. to ensure you always have water available.
- Pack some good-for-you quick snacks that are easily portable AND that are TSA-approved, if you are traveling by air. Some suggestions include: granola bars - KIND® and Kashi® are good brands, among others; pistachios, almonds, dried fruits, carrot sticks or baby carrots or other raw veggies, and/or apple slices. Having healthy snacks handy in your pocket or carry-on will help you ignore the temptations of fast-food and convenience stores.
- If meals are provided on your flight(s), when you book, try to order a vegetarian or special diet meal. These tend to be lower in carbs, sodium, and fat than the regular meals. If you forget to order a special meal in advance, then supplement the provided meal with some of your portable snacks so you're not

tempted to eat everything on your tray. Also, remember the refillable water bottle tip above!

- Remember to drink lots of water, particularly when you are flying, so you don't get dehydrated while traveling.
- In your hotel room, most hotels provide mini-refrigerators. If you are staying in the same hotel room for several days, consider stopping by a nearby grocery store for some healthy foods and snacks.   This will help you avoid the over-priced in-room snacks.
- If it is difficult or impossible to prepare food or snacks for yourself, try to order salads and other light and fresh menu items at restaurants. Commit to at lease one fresh and healthy meal each day. And watch your portions and consumption quantities: most of us don't eat appetizers and dinner salads and entrees and desserts during a single meal when we eat at home, so don't do it while you're traveling.

Exercise and Movement:

When you are sedentary for an extended amount of time, i.e., long flights, car rides, etc., you should make an effort to move every hour for at least 5 minutes or so. Walking up and down the airplane aisle or around the parking lot at a rest stop can make all the difference in your energy level when you arrive at your destination. Some easy-to-do stretches on an airplane are:

- Calf Raises
- Shoulder Stretch
- Spinal Twist
- Chest Stretch
- Tricep Stretch

If your hotel has a workout room, check out the hours and equipment in advance. Try to avoid the "rush hours" for working out so you have a better chance of getting on the equipment you want. Some hotels offer 24-hour fitness centers. If the hotel gym is not an option, here are some workout routines you can do in your hotel room with no equipment:

No-equipment Required Exercises in your Hotel Room:

Workout #1:

15 V- Ups, 15 Supermans, 14 V-Ups, 14 Supermans, 13,13,12,12 ………………..1,1

Workout #2:

3 Rounds:

1 Min Wall Sit

1 Min Plank Hold

1 Min Russian Twists

1 Min Superman Hold

Workout #3:

As Many Rounds as Possible in 8 Minutes:

10 V-Ups

20 Tuck Ins

30 Crunches

40 Supermans

50 Russian Twists

If your hotel does not offer a workout room, take a look at your surroundings. Is there a park or area where you could take a walk or a jog? Is there a shopping area that you could walk to and from to get a few items? Or, you could walk up and down a few flights of stairs if the weather is uncooperative or you're in an area that is not conducive to walking around outside. Also consider doing the in-room workout routines outlined above.

Daily Routines:

Sometimes when we travel, we ignore the daily personal routines we do when we're at home, like skincare, vitamins, and mental health. Practicing "total health" while you're traveling will help reduce travel-induced stress and also help you feel better.

- If you take vitamins or medications, pack them in travel containers and keep them with you in your carry-on bag. Maintain your routine for when you take your vitamins and medications.
- Pack travel-friendly sizes of your daily skincare, hair care, and other personal care items. Whatever you do while at home, be sure to do it while you're away. You don't want your skin or hair to suffer just because you're traveling.
- Regardless if your flight is short, cross country, or international, the circulated air inside the aircraft is dehydrating for both your body and your skin. To help you feel a bit fresher during flight, consider bringing along a face mist. There are several good brands available: Givenchy® Mist Me Gently; Kiehl's® In-Flight Refreshing Facial Mist; Clinique® Moisture Surge Face Spray, are some options, among others. Just be sure the bottle is 3 oz. or less so the TSA doesn't take it away from you!
- If you meditate or practice yoga or tai chi or other mental health activity while you're at home, schedule time to continue this practice while you're on the road. Keeping up with these routines should not undue restrictions on your trip, but rather will allow you to feel our best while you're busy on the road.

CHAPTER 8: MEAL PREP TIME SAVERS

As the saying goes, the only person who can save "Thursday you" from eating chips and salsa for dinner is "Sunday you", the plan-ahead person who takes just a couple of hours on Sunday to prepare healthy foods to get through the week. Make a plan to set aside an hour or two every Sunday to prep your meals and food for the coming week. You'll be glad you did!

Take time each weekend to do your grocery shopping and prepare your snacks and meals for the work week. Portion out your snacks into individual baggies and put any pre-made foods/snacks in sealed, portable containers so they're ready to go.

Tips for being prepared for your work week:

- Plan ahead – take a look at your calendar for the week to see if you have meetings, team lunches, business dinners, etc. and plan your meal prep accordingly
- Prepare your grocery list and stick to the list
- If you don't have proper portable food storage containers or baggies, add these to your shopping list
- Make full or large batches of recipes and either freeze the extra or store in airtight containers to eat on them during the week
- Wash, chop, and prepare most of your fruits and veggies for the week and store them in baggies or airtight containers
- Make the salad dressings and sauces, if applicable to your menu for the week
- For Monday's dinner, prep all ingredients (as much as possible) so all you have to do is mix, cook, and serve

EXERCISE GLOSSARY

Achilles Stretch

1. Start by placing your hands on the floor and lifting your hips as much as you can.
2. Keep your heels as far down as possible and straighten your legs as much as you can.
3. Walk your hands in closer to your feet for a deeper stretch.

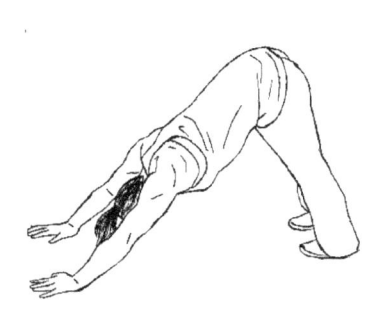

Alternating Lunges

1. Step out as far as you can with your right foot and bend both knees. Keep your chest upright.
2. Push off your right foot back to a stand.
3. Step out as far as you can with your left foot and bend both knees.
4. Push off your left foot back to a stand. That is one rep.

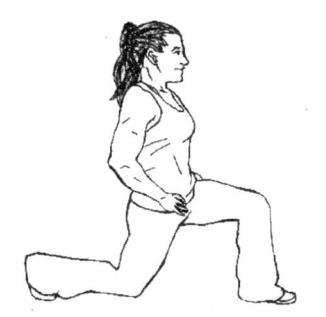

Bodyweight Squats

1. Start with your arms in front of you and your feet flat on the floor.
2. Sit your hips back keeping your heels pressed down and your chest up right.
3. Squat as low as you can and stand up to an upright position.

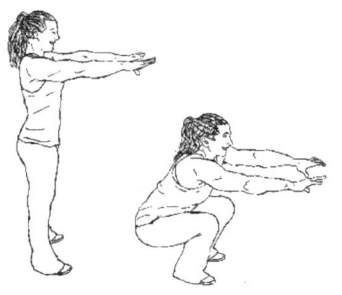

Calf Raises

1. Start by standing. Hold on to something stable (like your chair) for better balance.
2. Go as high as you can onto your toes and hold for 1 Second.
3. Go back down to flat feet and repeat.

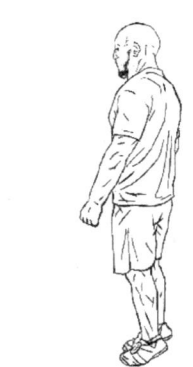

Cat Stretch

1. Start on your hands and knees and slide your hands out as far as you can.
2. Press your shoulders into the ground and hold.

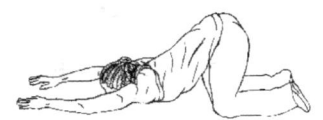

Chest Stretch

1. Start by sitting up tall or standing up.
2. Clasp hands behind your head.
3. Push your elbows as far back as you can and look up. Breath and hold.

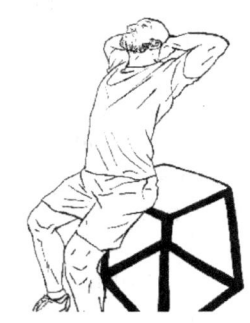

Chair Squats

1. Start by sitting on the edge of your chair with your arms out in front of your body.
2. Without using your hands, stand up by pressing your feet through the ground.
3. Sit back down and repeat.

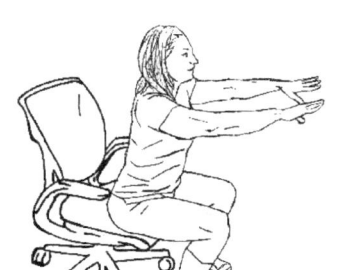

Cradle Stretch

1. Start by sitting at the edge of your chair and cross your right ankle over your left knee.
2. Lean forward and hold.
3. Switch legs and repeat. Be sure to breath for deeper stretching.

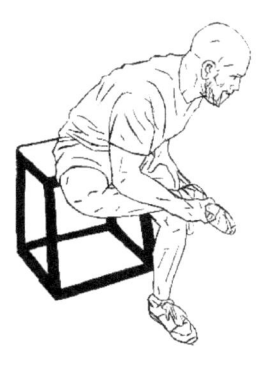

Crunches

1. Lie on your back and bend your knees.
2. Clasp your hands behind your head and lift your shoulders off the ground by squeezing your abdominals.
3. Relax back to a laying position and repeat.

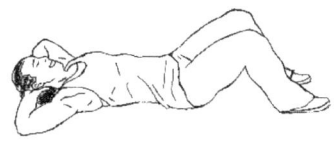

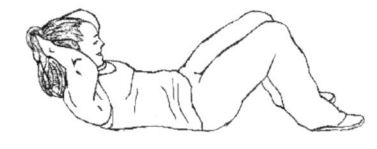

Desk Push Ups

1. Place your hands on the edge of your desk and walk your feet out from the desk.
2. Lower your body to the desk and push back up.

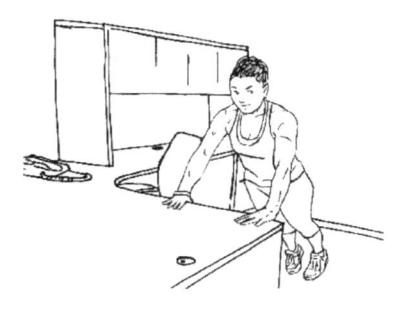

Figure 4 Stretch

1. Lie on your back and cross your right ankle over your left knee.
2. Pull your left knee into your body by grabbing the backside of your left knee.
3. Hold and breathe. Switch sides and repeat.

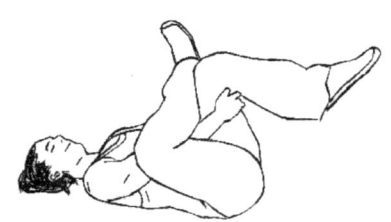

Hamstring Stretch (Sitting)

1. Sit at the edge of your chair and straighten one leg out in front of you. Lean forward until you feel a slight pull in the back of your leg.
2. Hold and breathe.
3. Switch legs and repeat.

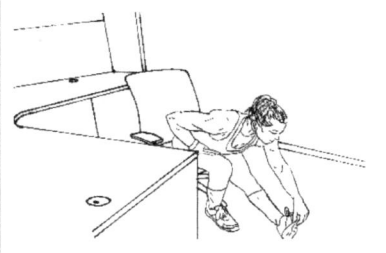

Hip Flexor/Hamstring Stretch

1. Start in the lunge position for a deep hip flexor stretch.
2. Rock back and straighten your front leg for a hamstring stretch.
3. Switch legs and repeat.

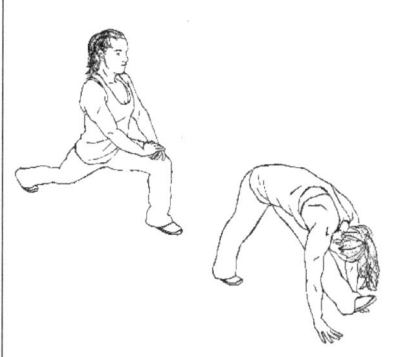

Jump Squats

1. Start by squatting as low as you can.
2. Then, jump as high as you can.
3. When you land the jump go back into a squat position and repeat.

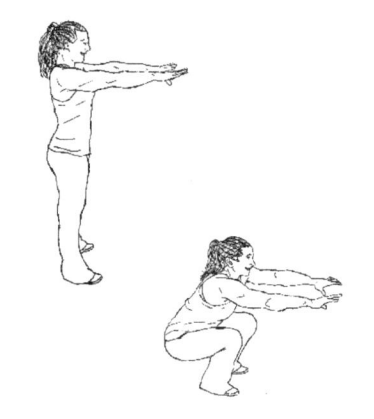

Jumping Jacks

1. Start in a standing position. Jump your feet out and swing your arms out to the side.
2. Jump your feet back together and bring your arms down to your side.
3. Repeat.

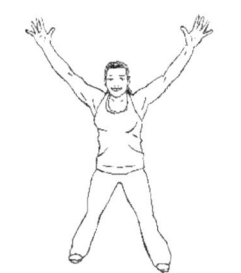

Knees Up

1. Start by standing up and lifting a knee as high as you can and then back down and switch legs.
2. This can be done in a marching motion or jogging in place motion based on ability.

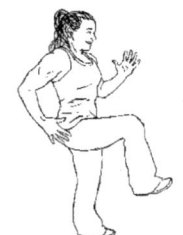

Lat Stretch

1. Sit tall and clasp your hands together overhead.
2. Lean to one side and hold. Switch sides and hold. Be sure breath deeply.

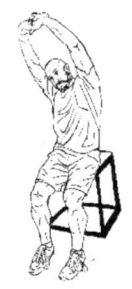

Lateral Raises

1. Start by sitting or standing with your arms down by your side.
2. Lift your arms out to the side until they are parallel to the ground.
3. Hold heavy objects in each hand to increase difficulty.
4. Relax arms down to the side and repeat.

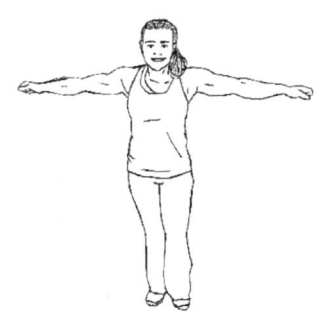

Leg Lifts

1. Start by lying down and placing hands underneath your hips (for added back support).
2. Keeping your legs straight, lift them off the ground as high as you can.
3. Lower your legs back down to the ground and repeat. **To modify, bend your knees.

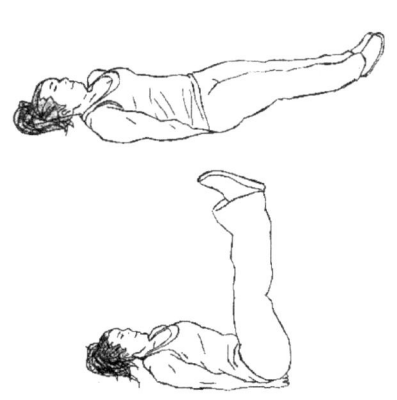

Leg Swings

1. Stand up and hold on to a chair or desk for support. Swing your leg back and forth as high as you can on each leg.
2. Switch legs and repeat.

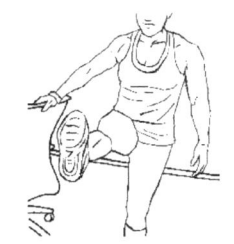

Modified Push Ups

1. Start by getting in a push up position, however, bend your knees to help support your body.
2. Keeping your body flat, bend your arms down and push back up.
3. Repeat.

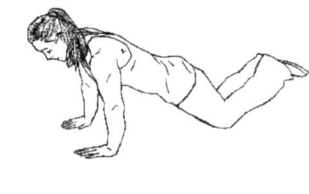

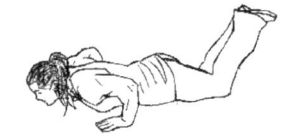

Pike Stretch

1. Sit in the pike position by stretching your legs out in front of your body.
2. Lean as far forward as you can and keep your legs straight.
3. Hold and breathe deeply.

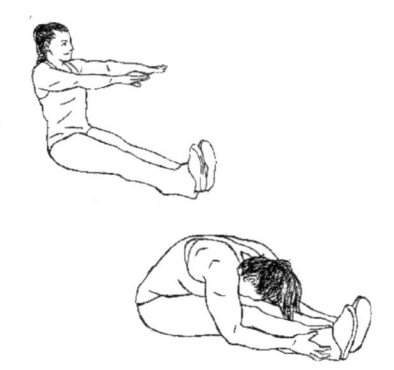

Plank Hold

1. Support your body on your elbows and your toes.
2. Be sure to keep your back flat (do not let your back arch).
3. Hold.

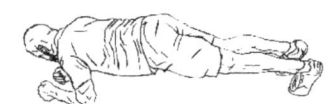

Push Ups

1. Support your body on your hand and toes.
2. Bend your arms and push back up. Be sure to
3. Repeat.

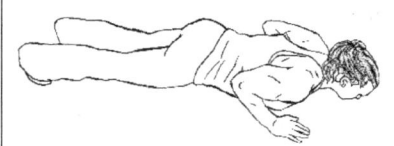

Russian Twists

1. Start by sitting, then lean back and lift your legs off the floor.
2. Twist side to side.
3. Hold a weight to increase intensity and difficulty.

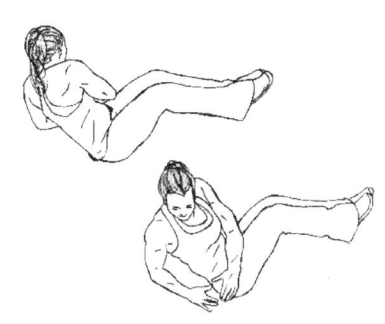

Seal Stretch

1. Lie on your stomach. Push you're your arms straight. To modify, support yourself on your elbows instead of hands.
2. Hold and breathe deeply.

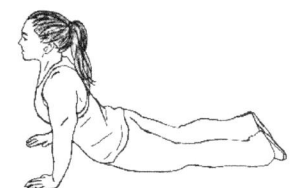

Shoulder Stretch

1. Cross your left arm over your body and use your right hand to your left elbow and pull your arm closer to your body.
2. Hold, relax, and breathe.

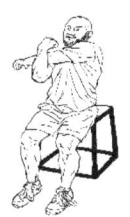

Small Arm Circles

1. Place your arms out to the side of your body.
2. Circle your arms in a small circular motion forward.
3. Switch directions and circle your arms backwards.

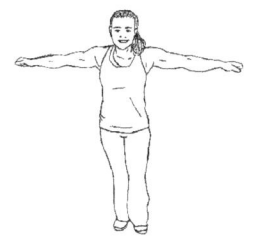

Spinal Twist

1. Sit tall in your chair. Twist backwards and use your arm to grab the back of your chair.
2. Switch sides.
3. Be sure to breathe deeply.

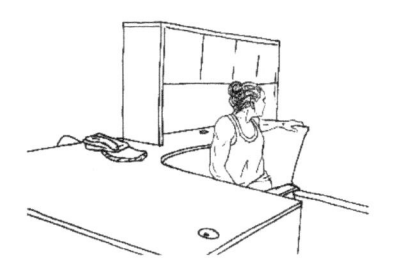

Standing Straddle Stretch

1. Stand up and step your legs out to the side.
2. Reach to your right leg and hold.
3. Reach to your left leg and hold.
4. Reach to the middle and hold.

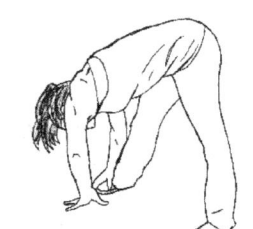

Straddle Stretch

1. Sit and straddle your legs as much as you can.
2. Reach to your right leg and hold.
3. Reach to your left leg and hold.
4. Reach to the middle and hold.

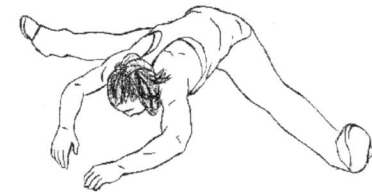

Supermans

1. Start by laying on your stomach.
2. Lift your arms and legs off the ground at the same time.
3. Hold for a second, relax, and repeat.

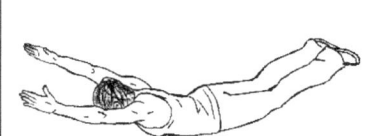

Tricep Dips

1. Start by sitting on a chair or a small step.
2. Keeping your hands planted, walk your feet out.
3. Bend your arms as much as you can and push back up. Repeat.

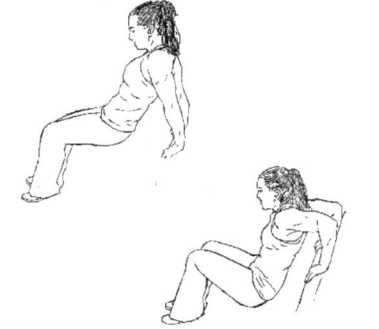

Tricep Stretch

1. Place one arm up over your head and bend it.
2. Using your other hand, grab your elbow and pull your arm back until you feel a stretch.
3. Hold and breathe.

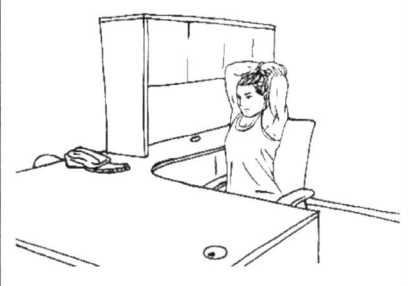

Trunk Twist

1. Sit in a pike position, bend one leg up, and cross your arm over your knee. Hold.
2. Switch sides and hold.

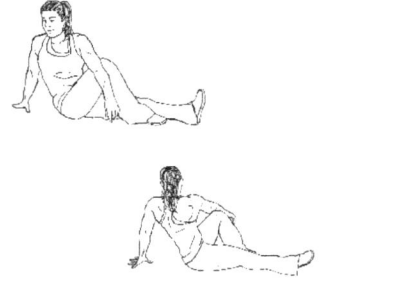

Tuck Ins

1. Lie on your back in a hollow body position.
2. Sit up and pull your knees into your chest simultaneously.
3. Relax back to the hollow body position and repeat.

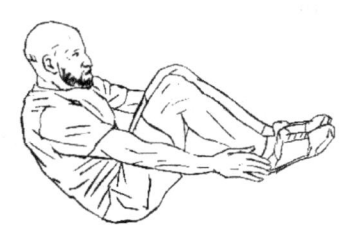

V-Ups

1. Lie on your back in a hollow body position.
2. Sit up and lift your legs up straight simultaneously.
3. Relax back to the hollow body position and repeat.

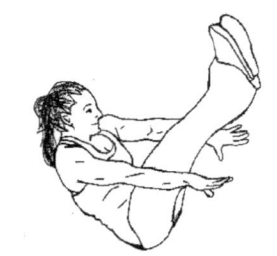

Wall Sit

1. Find a wall and lean your back against it.
2. Walk your feet out and bend your knees until your legs make a 90-degree angle.
3. Hold.

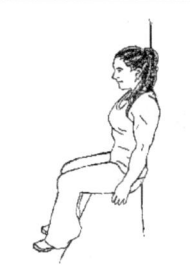

**Video demonstrations of all exercises can be found here:
http://astrongerworkplace.com/videos/

SOURCES

[1] Ewing Garber, C. (2011, July) *ACSM Issues New Recommendations on Quantity and Quality of Exercise.* Retrieved from: http://www.acsm.org/about-acsm/media-room/news-releases/2011/08/01/acsm-issues-new-recommendations-on-quantity-and-quality-of-exercise

[2] Bracko, M. (2011, August) *For All-Day Metabolism Boost, Try Interval Training.* Retrieved from: http://www.acsm.org/about-acsm/media-room/acsm-in-the-news/2011/08/01/for-all-day-metabolism-boost-try-interval-training

ABOUT: A STRONGER WORKPLACE

A Stronger Workplace, LLC is a corporate wellness company based in Atlanta, Georgia. A Stronger Workplace's mission is to help companies be more productive and more efficient by educating and motivating employees to live a healthier lifestyle. A Stronger Workplace's services include Lunch & Learns, Office Fitness Challenges, and Personal Training both onsite and online.

A Stronger Workplace, LLC was founded by Megan Hill in 2014. Megan is a graduate of Auburn University and earned both her Bachelor's and Master's Degrees in Health Promotion. She was also a member of the Auburn Gymnastics Team, Auburn Track & Field Team, as well as a former Pilot for the US Women's Bobsled Team. Megan is a Certified Exercise Physiologist by the American College of Sports Medicine. She uses her education along with athletic experiences to motivate and inspire health and wellness through A Stronger Workplace.

www.ingramcontent.com/pod-product-compliance
Lightning Source LLC
Chambersburg PA
CBHW070123290526
45789CB00005B/2122